Eat! Sleep! Meditate!

A Nurse's Guide to Health

Marva Riley, RN

Eat! Sleep! Meditate! A Nurse's Guide to Health

by Marva Riley

ISBN: 978-0-578-72807-0

Imprint: MarvaRiley

Cover Design: Susan Gulash of Gulash Graphics

Editing and Layout: Karen Yvonne Hamilton, Yesterday Press
www.yesterdaypress.com
Jupiter, Florida

DEDICATION

To my wonderful, amazing life partner and best friend Anthony Cutrera. Thank you for always inspiring me to think big. To reach beyond the stars. For believing in me when all I had was doubt. I look forward to umpteen more wonderful moments with us! To my precious children, Marlon & Marsha, I love you more than you can imagine. Thank you for my darling grandgirls Aria & Esti. One love!

Contents

INTRODUCTION

It is possible to be healthy at any age and without drugs. We are indeed what we eat. A body in motion does stay in motion. Sleep is vital for great health. Stress is one of the top causes of disease.

I have been a registered nurse for more than 22 years and have a passion for health and wellness. I love to tell true stories which are intended to help you and me attain and maintain great health. The steps to being healthy aren't rocket science. Anyone, if they want to, can attain and maintain great health, feel good in their bodies, be clear minded, be content and happy. You need only to make the decision today.

I hope my stories and tips will help you to be healthy; your health is your biggest wealth. The contents of this book are not intended to be used to diagnose or treat any medical conditions. I advise all my readers to consult their doctors before doing any changes that could affect your health.

In this book, I will show you how I healed myself of heart disease, depression, severe allergies, insomnia, and many more health issues using a wholistic[1] approach and without drugs. I will show you how to grow older, healthy, happy, and strong. Just follow my guidelines and you will experience health beyond your wildest imaginations.

Let's get started!

---

[1] 'Wholistic': A Natural Evolution Of 'Holistic' The 'w' brings the meaning full circle. https://www.merriam-webster.com/words-at-play/wholistic-word-origin-and-use

RECOGNIZING THE BRAINWASH

I had been frail for most of my life. As a child, I experienced frequent headaches and never had much energy. During my teenage life, I had heavy menstrual periods with unbearable pain and cramps, bleeding in between my period and always low on energy. At the age of 15, the doctor placed me on birth control pills to help regulate the menstrual bleeding.

At the age of 30, I suddenly became allergic to fish and seafood. The allergy was so severe that I was unable to be in a room, or for that matter, any building where fish and seafood were being stored or prepared. Even going to the supermarket was a challenge. I always carried an epinephrine pen with me wherever I went. I continued to cheat and eat sardines, shrimp, and other kinds of seafood, but my doctor told me on one of my visits to choose life or fish. It was that serious. There were multiple visits to the emergency room where I presented with swelling of my entire body, tongue, and throat, hives and shortness of breath.

Visits to any restaurants or eateries involved extensive interviews to ascertain if there was a possibility of cross contamination of my food with fish or seafood. Waiters were usually quite frustrated and looked at me as if I had two heads. I began to announce upfront to them that I was severely allergic to fish and seafood and was not trying to be difficult.

It was about this age that I started experiencing other health challenges like sinusitis, allergic rhinitis, headaches, and migraines. This led to antihistamine drugs, ibuprofen, and frequent visits to the doctor who would often prescribe steroids, antihistamines, cough drugs, among others. The allergy drugs worked for a while, then they stopped. Sometimes I was placed on multiple allergy drugs in hopes of controlling the sneezing, coughing, headaches, runny nose, chest and nasal congestion, maddening headaches and painful sinuses.

About the age of 40, I started having periods of forgetfulness and confusion. At that time I worked as a critical care nurse and I remember being very afraid that I would forget the protocol for cardiac resuscitation if my patient coded blue or if it was my turn to respond to a code blue anywhere else in the hospital. I recall leaving my husband and children at one of the kids' soccer games, heading to the clinic to see my doctor about this confusion and forgetfulness I was experiencing along with lightheadedness, dizziness, and a general malaise or low energy. Shortly after getting into my car, I forgot where I was going, although I had been to that place multiple times before. I pulled over into a vacant lot and just sat in my car until things started coming back to me.

A CT scan and MRI were done along with multiple blood tests including B12 level. They all came back negative. My primary doctor told me that I was in pre-menopause and was experiencing menopausal depression. I was promptly placed on Lexapro, an antidepressant which did help me to feel less hopeless but was not the answer to my many fears and questions. This was a Band-Aid used to cover up a deeper, and more serious issue. But, isn't this what many doctors do? They prescribe drugs that do not heal, that never cure but mask the symptoms of the deeper issues in our bodies, our minds, and our spirits. Why was I feeling this way? What was happening to me? I felt old, helpless.

Within a couple of years, things escalated, and I began to experience dizziness, lightheadedness, severe shortness of breath, along with very low energy to the point where I could only walk short distances in my own house without having to sit, rest, and take a breath. I was stubborn, ignorant, and perhaps downright stupid because not only did I not go to the emergency room, I didn't go to see my doctor. And yes, I was at this time a registered nurse working in critical care. It is said that doctors and nurses take care of everybody first and themselves last. Yes, I am embarrassed to say that was me. If my husband and children had a finger pain, I would rush them to the doctor, but here I was feeling like I was dying, even with much cajoling from my husband, still I refused to take any steps to help myself. Yes, dumb!

Finally, after experiencing much dyspnea (difficult or labored respiration) climbing stairs, I went to see my doctor. His nurse practitioner attended to me. She ordered an EKG because by now I was having serious palpitations, lightheadedness, dizziness and was so weak I could hardly care for myself. The EKG showed ventricular tachycardia of up to 12 beats. She immediately called a cardiologist and instructed me to head over to see him at once.

The echocardiogram revealed that I had cardiomyopathy of unknown etiology with ejection fraction of 35% and ventricular tachycardia. In essence, this meant that my heart muscles were very weak and functioning at 35% (60% to 100% is considered normal). The reason for the weak heart muscles were unknown and this weak heart muscle led to life threatening irregular heartbeats. Drugs were the treatment of choice, beta blockers and aspirin. My cardiologist had warned me of the main side effects of beta blockers: dizziness, weakness, fatigue, and drowsiness to name a few. These symptoms, which I was already experiencing, intensified to the point where he had to quickly switch drugs to ace inhibitors, another category of drugs used to treat patients with heart failure or potential heart failure; this didn't make the symptoms any less. I felt like I was dying. My cardiologist told me that a heart transplant was my only hope as I could not tolerate the more conventional treatments.

On many occasions I had to leave work due to severe palpitation or just plain feeling sick. One of the nurses I worked with recommended that I see an electrophysiologist that she was familiar with and was highly recommended. An electrophysiologist is a medical doctor who specializes in the electrical function of the heart. Upon seeing him, he informed me that my weak heart muscles led to the irregular heartbeat and that the other doctor was treating me as if the irregular heartbeats had led to the weak heart muscles.

One week later, he performed a cardiac ablation which he stated would cure me of this condition. This procedure, he explained, is used to terminate faulty electrical pathways from areas of my heart that were causing the irregular heartbeats or arrhythmias called Ventricular Tachycardia. Ventricular Tachycardia is a heart condition that causes the ventricles or lower chambers of the heart to beat rapidly. If this condition is not treated quickly and effectively, it can lead to a more serious condition called Ventricular Fibrillation where the lower chambers of the heart (ventricles) contract very rapidly in an uncoordinated manner. This could lead to sudden death due to cardiac arrest. At my 2-week follow up visit, he told me to flush all my heart pills down the toilet, including the aspirin. He instructed me to start walking every day, cut out coffee and green tea due to their caffeine content, eat healthy, and decrease my stress level.

He did not have to tell me this more than once. I immediately started walking 30 minutes every day, and I have never turned back to my old unhealthy way of living.

I started to read a bit about healthy living and alternatives to “medications” where I bumped into a book written by Kevin Trudeau. I read it and started practicing a few of his teachings, such as getting at least 30 minutes of exercise in the sun each day. Researchers have proven that a deficiency in vitamin D, which we get from the sun, leads to many diseases and disorders. The book also suggested the use of ice or heat to relieve pain instead of pain pills. Trudeau also recommended getting eight hours or more of sleep every night and eating mostly plant-based foods and fewer meats. But, I still didn't quite get it.

Meat was such an integral part of my culture and upbringing. I didn't feel that I could ever *not* eat meat for dinner and lunch every day. Also, I bought into the brainwash, although I didn't know it was a brainwash at the time. The brainwash that protein was vital to good health and that meat/animal products, eggs, fish and seafood were the number one source or best source of proteins. I bought into the brainwash that milk, cheese, yogurt, chicken, beef, eggs, pork (the so-called white meat) should make up a large portion of all our meals. I adopted what I thought was a healthy way of eating. That is 50% meat protein, 10% vegetables, rice, wheat bread, and I felt very pleased with myself that I was eating healthy. Overall, I was feeling better; however, the allergies continued and even worsened over time.

Fast forward to 2012. I was 50 years old. I had been through two traumatic divorces within four years. I was stressed, overworked, and unhappy. There were many questions and no answers. I decided to pray, meditate, and read my Bible. I was searching for answers.

THE HEALING BEGINS

In one year, I read the Bible twice from Genesis to Revelation. The more I read, the more questions I had. Many nights were spent in tears on my knees seeking God's guidance and direction. Seeking answers to my many whys. Seeking comfort. Longing for peace. Longing to feel loved. Longing...

As I spent hours by myself, turning within, I discovered that the peace I so longed for was there, deep within my being. That the God I felt had abandoned me was there, there all along, but I was unaware of that. I became aware that the love I longed for, I already had, God's love was me. I became aware that for anyone to love me purely and unconditionally, I needed to love myself purely and unconditionally, the way God loves me. I discovered in my quiet moments with God that I didn't need to work to earn His love. God loves me just as I am. The healing had begun!

After many unsuccessful dating experiences, I decided to put that pursuit on hold and just enjoy myself by myself. I loved the Arts: dancing, movies, plays, concerts etc. I decided I would explore all of these by myself. At this time all my girlfriends had found men and were busy with their lives, so I started venturing out by myself. At first, it was frightening. My first marriage was at the age of nineteen to my first boyfriend. That lasted for over twenty-five years. I had never lived on my own. Then shortly after that marriage ended, I married again. I never knew what living by myself felt like. I never knew what it was like to go to the movies or a play, let alone a night club by myself. So that's what I mean when I say it was frightening. I recall the first time I went to a sports bar by myself; I spilled the glass of Coca-Cola in my lap. I quietly tiptoed out, headed home, and had a nice big long laugh. That did not deter me though. The next Friday I was at a lounge shaking my booty. I intended to live my life to the fullest with or without a man. The healing continued!

Not too long after, on a beautiful Friday night, after completing a long twelve-hour shift at the hospital, I headed home to a lonely house. I was off for the long weekend, so I decided to put on my red dress and my high heels, get myself all dolled up, and hit the road. I headed to *Mangoes* in Fort Lauderdale to listen to some live music, drink Coca-Cola and shake my booty a bit. Whilst standing at the back of the bar, a handsome gentleman walked up to me, asked for a dance, and the rest is history. That became the beginning of a wonderful partnership, one that would lead me to a healthier and happier way of life. The healing continues!

As a wise woman should, I invited my new man to dinner, cooking my favorite Jamaican dishes of curried goat, jerk chicken, rice 'n' peas and a salad with my favorite Vidalia onion dressing. I planned to impress the shirt off his back. I was most disappointed to hear him say that he was not into meat much and would only eat the salad minus the dressing. "I will just have a little olive oil with vinegar," he said. I was fit to be tied but tried my best to hide it.

Anthony and I met in August 2012. By November of the same year, I started feeling very ill. It seemed I was becoming severely allergic to everything including water. But how could it be? No one is ever allergic to everything! Well, I was. The only things that I could consume that did not make me sick were Publix purified water and boniato sweet potato. Everything that I ate or touched caused me to experience shortness of breath, severe headaches, severe dry eyes, chest tightness, hives and rash with pustules, swollen lips and eyelids, joint pain, unsteady gait, dizziness, and lightheadedness. Was I dying? Not only was I severely allergic to foods, but I was also allergic to toothpaste, lotions, deodorants, hair products, cleaning products, and soaps.

I recalled having a patient with a similar situation who had been hospitalized on many occasions with anaphylaxis, a severe and potentially life-threatening allergic reaction, requiring intubation, steroids and antihistamines for extensive periods to save her life. After multiple admissions, with the doctors not knowing the cause of her illness,, she was treated as if she made up her symptoms, like she had Munchausen Syndrome, although we nurses could clearly see the swelling of her body, the rash all over, the swelling of her tongue. The steroids used to treat this patient led to her later diagnoses of insulin dependent diabetes and subsequent kidney injury. One drug after the other was added to her regimen.

I knew that this was not the way I wanted to be treated but didn't know what my alternatives were. Within weeks, I had lost twenty pounds and dropped from a size eight to size zero and felt like I was dying. I did not go to the emergency room because I knew the treatment would have been steroids and Benadryl, Band-Aids. An allergy test done by a specialist revealed that I was allergic to everything they tested for except roaches. I refused her offer of steroids and Benadryl.

I had just started a new job as a hospice case manager when I ran into a medical doctor whom I knew from a previous hospital where I worked as a critical care nurse. He inquired of my health, commenting that I looked like sh...t. He then introduced me to an alternative eastern medical treatment protocol called NAET which he told me is used for treating and curing allergies. He had tried it himself and completely "cured" of his many allergies and recommended I try it. NAET is Nambudripad's Allergy Elimination Techniques. It is a non-invasive, drug free treatment methodology used to treat allergy related illnesses. NAET is usually practiced by acupuncturists and chiropractors. My medical doctor however offered this treatment protocol because he had proven that it worked.

The next six months would find me in the office of an acupuncturist who was also a NAET practitioner. Her finding confirmed that I was allergic to "everything". My first NAET treatment helped, so that for the next two weeks, I could safely eat boniato sweet potatoes and Publix purified water without any adverse reaction. One by one I was treated for allergy to one food at a time, toiletries, and eventually even for psychological issues. Some foods like sardines required six or more treatments. As I was treated and cleared of these allergens, I started feeling better, regaining some weight, and the symptoms gradually resolved. It was a long and hard road. I spent hundreds of dollars for treatments because at the time I was between jobs and had no insurance coverage. Baking soda served as my toothpaste, mouthwash, dish detergent, laundry soap, bath soap, antiperspirant and hair shampoo. Anything else led to severe allergic reactions including dizziness, lightheadedness, and imbalance.

At this critical time, I craved the support of my new life partner. 'Support' had a certain 'look' for me, and I didn't feel like Anthony was being supportive as he kept emphasizing that this illness was the best thing that had ever happened to me. This, he said had forced my body into a fast, and that this fast was what was going to lead to my healing. I was also not pleased that he did not encourage my constant desire to talk about what was ailing me, how bad I was feeling, how sick I felt and so on. His constant advice was that I should 'ignore' the 'feelings'. He also encouraged me to take my mind off how I felt and focus on how I wanted to feel. All of this did not make sense to me. I had never heard any such things before. Feeling hurt, I seethed with resentment towards him.

My twenty plus years of nursing practice made me very aware that western medicine offered no cure but were Band-Aids for symptoms. Drugs and more drugs were the standard protocol for all that ails. I was convinced that there had to be another way other than drugs. This led to numerous researches. I eventually turned to the Internet, books, acupuncturists, herbalists, chiropractors. I was hungry for answers. For a cure to my many illnesses. Everything pointed to nutrition and lifestyle.

I read hundreds of testimonials from people who had healed themselves of all kinds of diseases and disorders through homeopathy, eastern medicine, herbs, and overall lifestyle changes. Everything pointed to wholistic healing through lifestyle changes. Out of desperation I decided to try this. This led to a radical change from my current diet to a plant-based diet/nutrition. Before this, I had heard Dr Oz say that one could start by doing one meatless day per week, then gradually increase the days, and that's how I began. This process took about two months. It was not easy. I fell back many times. Eventually, I was meatless. Immediately I started to feel like a new person. Joint pains and depression lessened. Sleep came easier and lasted longer. I started feeling energized and alive. I began to heal.

At that same time, I started working on my spiritual life by spending at least two hours per day by myself in quietness or meditation/prayer as some call it. As I became more comfortable with my own company, I felt more and more at peace, content, settled and happy. This, I believe is what the Christian Bible meant by "the peace that surpasses all understanding."

Gratitude journaling became a way of life for me. It helped me to focus on the good things and good times in my life. Much time was spent at the beach, by a pond or some large body of water where I felt closest to God.

Realizing that the body, soul, and spirit work together to bring wholeness and harmony, I ventured on a consistent exercise regimen. I spent four days per week at the gym where I met new people, including a 90-year-old gentleman who inspired me so much. He told me that he went skydiving for his 90th birthday, had a girlfriend who was sixty years old, spent two hours at the gym daily, and rode a motorbike as a hobby.

I was the only female in the weight room and the men there would constantly praise and inspire me. I was looking hot and I knew it. This sent my confidence through the roof. Although walking was my favorite exercise and is certainly known to be the best form of exercise, I did so enjoy the gym and the social life I had there.

My healthier lifestyle led to better, longer sleep. I woke up in the mornings feeling rested and ready to face the challenges of the day. I adopted the healthy habit of going to bed at 9:30 to 10 pm every night and getting up at 5 am on workdays and 6:30 am on off days. It is during sleep time at night that our bodies heal and repair themselves. So, it's vital that we get enough rest every night if we want to be healthy and stay healthy. The mind and spirit also need adequate night rest to perform at its optimal.

As I continued to study, research, and ask questions, I began to learn about the healing virtues of plants, herbs. I also learned of the many negative effects of meat and any animal by-products. I began to learn that plant-based eaters have fewer diseases than carnivores.

My life was changing for the better. I was feeling the best I had ever felt. I became energetic and strong as my body healed itself with the help of good nutrition, decreased stress, adequate sleep, moderate exercise, prayer and meditation as a way of life.

There are no quick fixes or shortcuts to health. It takes work and dedication. Some people like to ask me, "What can I take to get rid of hot flashes, or what can I take to get rid of arthritis?" There is no one thing to take to get rid of a health issue.

Health is a lifestyle!

Healing takes discipline.

There is no quick fix.

I would like to share a few tips, recipes, guidelines that have led to my healthy way of living, healthy body, mind and spirit. They work for me, and I feel that they'll work for you as well.

CHOOSING A LIFESTYLE

Some of my favorite spices and herbs are

- ginger root
- turmeric root
- fresh onion
- fresh scallions
- fresh garlic bulb
- fresh thyme
- fresh rosemary
- any fresh mint
- fennel seeds
- caraway seeds
- crushed red peppers
- fresh clove buds which I grind myself
- whole pimento which I grind myself

These are natural, tasty, inexpensive, nutritious, and unprocessed.

Every one of the above spices and herbs are very good at aiding in proper digestion. They do not overpower the natural flavors of whatever we cook but enhance them.

Since I'm a plant-based eater, all my dinners incorporate beans. One could say that beans and peas are my meat. Dried beans have a long shelf life, are inexpensive and loaded with complex carbohydrates, protein, calcium, iron, fiber, vitamin C, magnesium, sodium, potassium, copper, manganese, zinc, folate, and phosphorus to name a few. Beans are one of the least expensive sources of protein, especially when compared to meat. Besides, we do not need nearly as much protein as the meat industry touts. We need fresh vegetables and fresh fruits.

Neither do we need to eat meat to live a long, healthy life. I once heard an older man who'd built his business from scratch and was now quite wealthy but was plagued with chronic illnesses state, "I was much healthier when I was poor." His point was that he ate much less meat when he was poor because he could not afford to eat a lot of meat. Once he started making money, he began eating "the king's diet," steak, seafood, fish, the finest pork chops, the best-dressed chicken, etc.

This reminds me of the story in the Christian Bible of Daniel and his friends. They were taken from their homeland to be trained forcibly for the king's exclusive service (I paraphrase). Daniel and his friends were plant-based eaters and wanted nothing to do with the king's rich [meaty] diet. They begged their trainer to allow them to eat fruits, vegetables, nuts, and grains during a period. Plant-based foods. The agreement was that if they were not stronger or as strong as the other young men, then they would eat from the king's table. After the time had elapsed, Daniel and his friends were stronger, more clear-minded, and more physically appealing than their peers. If only we Christians would learn from Daniel and the Hebrew boys, we would be healthier and stronger, not just physically, but emotionally, spiritually and psychologically. Their diet was not just during a fast as some churches practice; it was a lifestyle.

Since you're reading this book I know it's safe for me to assume that there is an interest in your health. That is not the norm, and so I commend you on that. Every one of us needs to take an interest in our health. If we don't, who will? The drug companies want us sick. How else could they be one of the richest businesses on earth? The hospitals, clinics, nursing homes and rehabilitation centers, dialysis centers want us sick.

How else could they make the millions they do if we didn't have cancer, heart diseases, diabetes, kidney failures?

We are in the middle of the coronavirus pandemic and many hospitals, clinics, outpatient centers and other healthcare-related businesses have laid off thousands of their workers. How could this be, you may ask. It's because the unhealthy are not doing elective surgeries and procedures which is one of the number one income for this industry. Many drug companies are working around the clock to produce a vaccine for this coronavirus. Of course, they are, there are billions of dollars to be made for the company that comes up with this vaccine. Whereas the scientists are saying that it could take up to 18 months to create a vaccine, the president of the United States is bent on having one before the end of the year. Of course, he's bent on making this happen, not, in my opinion, because he cares about me or you or anyone, but because it's an election year, and he must win no matter if this vaccine is safe or not.

In my opinion, no vaccine is safe. Speaking of vaccines, the worst respiratory sickness I have ever had was after I was forced to take the influenza vaccine when I worked in a nursing home over 20 years ago. Since then, I have fought hospitals tooth and nail every flu season as they threaten those of us who decline the vaccine. Many healthcare facilities are mandating it, and one cannot work there if one has not been vaccinated. I strongly encourage you to read the side effects of the flu vaccine. If you do, you would, like me, adamantly refuse to have that poison in your bodies.

The doctors and yes, we nurses, want us sick. How else could any doctor make $200,000 or more per year, and how could nurses and other healthcare workers be the top paid professionals in the United States? If the hospital census is low, the staff is sent home without pay unless we have paid time off, and when the PTO is finished, we are sent home or canceled without pay. No pay, no money, no money, and we can't live in our nice houses, drive nice cars, and take nice vacations. Yes, unfortunately, we do like it when the census is high so we can have a job. Doesn't that add up to us wanting you to be sick? Think about that. Where am I going with this? We must take responsibility for our health because no one else will.

I strongly advise everyone to have a trusted relative or friend to be your advocate when you go to the doctor, a clinic, a long-term care facility, rehabilitation center, or the hospital. Be sure to have your power of attorney and health care surrogate/health care proxy/living will legal documents prepared now. Make a copy and keep it with you all the time. Discuss your desires and wishes including end of life decisions with your healthcare surrogate and be sure to give them a copy of these documents.

Due to the HIPPA law[2], your loved ones may not be able to get any information about your health condition from the healthcare team if they do not have a legal document stating that they can. That's where the aforementioned legal documents come in handy and important. Someone you want will be able to speak and advocate for you if you can't do so or are unable to make decisions for yourself. Sometimes we just need another set of eyes and ears even when we're still competent. Illnesses make us very anxious and unable to think clearly in a crisis or emergency.

Health is a lifestyle. Step by step. Believe me when I say that you will fall. The importance is to get up and keep trying, persevere.

Like a baby, you'll fall. When the baby falls, he/she gets up and tries again. Not all babies learn at the same time or the same speed. Slow and steady wins the race is what they say. Health, however, is not a race, it's a journey.

---

[2] The Health Insurance Portability and Accountability Act of 1996 (HIPAA) is a federal law that required the creation of national standards to protect sensitive patient health information from being disclosed without the patient's consent or knowledge.

HEALTHY HABITS

For our entire life, we'll be working on healthy habits and a healthy lifestyle which encompasses

- Nutritious, primarily plant-based eating
- Moderate exercise. Walking is man's best medicine, says Hippocrates who is called the father of western medicine.
- Let's get good sleep. I do believe, and I have proven, that we do need a minimum of 7 to 8 hours of sound sleep. Don't let anyone tell you otherwise.
- Relax. Decrease your stress level.
- Pray, be still, meditate regularly.
- Have fun. Find a hobby, something to do that gives you joy. Pray.
- Guard your mind. The TV, Internet and technology clamor for our mind and attention. Be in charge of your mind. Don't allow them to take charge of your mind.
- Live a simple lifestyle as best as you can. Some of us are more prone to anxiety, worry, and excessive stress. Those are the ones that need to be more diligent about guarding your minds against negativity and too much media. Such a person can benefit from a healthy

routine like going to bed at the same time each night and waking up at the same time every morning.. Such persons need to eat healthy balanced meals and get regular exercise. They also need "me" time, time alone in quietness and meditation.

- Develop a hobby and find things to do that give you pleasure. Write a book. Do some gardening. Visit the sick. Volunteer to read to sick children. Adopt a pet.

Why is good nutrition important?

Good nutrition and adequate hydration lead to a healthier you. We are what we eat. As we eat, digestion starts in the mouth while we chew and swallow. Eventually, whatever we eat ends up in our bloodstream and is taken to the various organs of our body. So, if we eat healthy foods, that is what our organs are getting. If we eat unhealthy foods like burgers, bread, cookies, crackers, hot dogs, excess sugar, soda pop, sweetened juices, processed foods, excess animal products, this is what we are feeding our organs. Poor diet leads to diseases such as heart disease, diabetes, hypertension, kidney diseases, obesity, asthma, depression, sleep disorder, and constipation, potentially resulting in a shortened life span. Healthy eating will likely lead to vibrant disease-free living.

A plant-based diet, in my opinion, based on my personal experience and according to much research, is the healthiest. All the nutrients our body requires to stay healthy and strong are in fruits, vegetables, nuts, grains, beans, and peas. It is recommended that one takes vitamin B12 supplements or eat foods fortified with B12 as to date there is apparently no evidence that B12 exists in a plant-based diet. A plant-based diet nourishes and helps our bodies to heal and repair themselves. A plant-based diet also helps our body to ward off diseases and illnesses as it improves our immunity. We need to teach our children how to eat healthy by introducing them to fruits, vegetables, nuts, grains, legumes, and water as babies.

They need to see the family eating healthy. Children learn what they live and will carry this good habit into adulthood.

Some have asked, is it possible to eat healthy on a low income, on a low budget? My answer is yes! Junk is not cheap. Meat, fish, eggs, cheese, milk, bread, cake, cookies, crackers, soda, and sweet drinks are not cheap. Eating out at fast food joints is not cheap. I see plenty of fast food places, restaurants, and grocery stores everywhere, and they are always packed.

I know many fruits are quite expensive off season. But, if we eat them during the season, we'll pay much less. Many healthy vegetables are quite reasonably priced.

- Cabbage, carrots, kale and collards when in season can be quite affordable.
- Beans and peas are affordable.
- Brown rice is reasonable.
- Onion and garlic are inexpensive and filling.
- Tomatoes go on sale during its season.
- Lemon and lime are very high in vitamin C and other nutrients. They don't cost too much.
- Bananas are fairly affordable and are rich in minerals and other nutrients.
- Oatmeal is affordable, healthy, and a great option for breakfast.

We can also save money on food by eating fewer quantities. Buy fruits, vegetables, grains, nuts, beans when they're on sale and when they're in season. I eat sweet potatoes during the fall because they are in abundance and much cheaper. Right now, grapes are $3.49 per pound. I will not be eating that unless they go on a good sale. Right now, apples are $.98 per pound and bananas $.59 per pound. I eat them when they are on sale. Stay away from canned fruits and vegetables. They are packed with unlisted additives, sodium, sugar, and preservatives which are bad for your health.

Plant Based Eating

I suggest that you gradually change to a plant-based diet. I started by eliminating all meats and animal products including fish from my diet one day per week for one month. Then I increased it to two days per week for one month and so on until I was completely meatless with no animal products including milk, cheese, fish, seafood. It is often taught that we need animal products for protein and calcium, but that is not true.

All the protein and calcium that our body needs to be healthy and strong are available in

- Beans
- Peas
- Lentils
- Nuts
- Seeds
- Grains (amaranth, seaweeds)
- Green leafy vegetable (collards, turnip, spinach)
- Oranges (rich in calcium)
- Blackberries (rich in calcium)
- Blackstrap molasses (loaded with calcium).

I recall telling a physician that I had switched to plant-based eating and his main concern was that I would not be getting my calcium. I had to laugh because clearly he had not done many studies on food and nutrition, or he would be well aware that there are many calcium and protein rich plants. One does not need milk to get an adequate amount of these nutrients. Vitamin B12 does not have to come from beef consumption.

Plant-based eaters can take B12 supplements instead of eating beef. My Vegan friends eat B12 fortified foods.

Millions of chickens, cows, pigs, goats, turkeys, sheep, fish, and other seafood are bred daily for the sole purpose of being slaughtered for food. These animals, like us, get sick with various illnesses and infections. They too are being given numerous drugs to keep them just healthy enough to be slaughtered and packaged for the meat department and subsequently end up on our plates. We are told to eat meat from animals that are grass-fed, suggesting that it is healthier, but, I'm sure that you, like me, have wondered what is in that grass? What chemical was used to spray the grass that the animals eat, that we eventually eat?

Most animals whose meats we eat are fed with processed animal feed made from genetically modified corn and other genetically modified grains. Why do humans need to drink cow's milk or any other milk for that matter? Humans should be drinking human milk as babies, not milk from cows, sheep, or any other animals. Cheese is loaded with all kinds of preservatives and loads of salt which are not conducive to good health. Have you thought about the negative effects that processed meat have on our health? Cancer is one of the main causes of death in the world today. Researchers have linked processed meat to cancer. Why do we continue to eat bacon, salami, hot dogs, ham, sausages?

The environment is being severely affected by the amount of waste being disposed of from cultivated animals bred solely for consumption. We are dying from diseases that come from animal products. You've heard of the mad cow disease, right?

Being a plant-based eater does not mean eating a boring salad every day. One can be quite creative with salads by adding different nuts like walnut, almond, pecan and or boiled wild rice, brown or black rice, quinoa, barley, corn, spelt and teff. Steamed or cooked vegetables are healthy and very tasty. With time, you will acquire the individual delicious taste of vegetables. Steamed vegetables can be spiced up with onions, garlic, tomatoes, peppers, and some seasoning salt or seasalt, just like we would spice up the meats we eat.

Remember, meats by themselves have no taste without some salt, peppers, and spices. Well, it's the same way with vegetables. We need to spice them up to make them enjoyable and tasty.

I will be sharing some tasty plant-based recipes with you later in this book. Keep on reading.

I want to highlight that plant-based eating is not the same as vegan eating. As a plant-based eater, I stay away from unhealthy junk food like cookies, crackers, and bread. I prepare my vegetables fresh, cooking my beans and peas from scratch, and eating fresh as opposed to canned or frozen fruits or vegetables. These I call *live foods*. Processed foods I call *dead foods* with little to no real nutrients. Many vegans that I know do not eat healthy but eat processed dead foods, lots of sugar and salt. As a plant-based eater you will eat primarily fresh vegetables and fresh fruits, not frozen or canned. You will eat peas and beans cooked from scratch, and healthy nuts like almonds, pecans, walnuts, Brazilian nuts, and cashew nuts.

I am aware that many pieces of research have shown that meat-eaters are more likely to die from chronic diseases including heart disease, diabetes, stroke and other obesity related diseases.

The number one killer in the United States is heart disease. Heart diseases are mainly a result of obesity. Obesity is a direct result of overeating, eating the wrong types of foods, insufficient exercise, insufficient sleep, and excess stress. Heart diseases lead to high blood pressure, plaque formation in the arteries and veins, stroke, heart attacks, and circulation problems. Heart diseases can be prevented or reversed by adopting a plant-based diet along with moderate exercise like walking for 30 minutes at least four days per week. It can be prevented or reversed by getting 8 hours of good sleep per night and reducing our stress levels.

Another killer is diabetes. Diabetes is a debilitating disease that affects billions around the world. Diabetes can be reversed or prevented by adopting the same healthy lifestyle I mentioned before. Insulin and diabetes drugs are Band-Aids. The issue is the lifestyle. Change the lifestyle, get rid of the disease. I know several people who have been able to get off all drugs for cholesterol, hypertension, chronic pain, arthritis, diabetes and coronary heart/coronary artery disease by adopting a plant-based healthy diet, walking 30 minutes per day for 4 days per week, getting adequate sleep and decreasing stress levels. Yes, it's possible for them, for me, and for you as well.

If one chooses to eat meat/flesh, small portions would be best. After all, a little bit of poison is less likely to kill than a lot of poison. As of now, there is no evidence that vitamin B12 is available in plants. It may be, but since we are a society of evidence-based practice, it is probably a good practice to include a vitamin B12 supplement in our dietary regimen. All other nutrients necessary for healthy living are readily available in the right proportions in a plant-based diet.

Many have told me that they can't give up flesh. I too felt that way until death knocked on my door. Until arthritis and inflammation left me almost paralyzed. Until heart disease left me feeling like I had one foot in the grave and one out. I too felt like I couldn't give up flesh until no drug that was given to me worked, and I was sure that death was just around the corner. Until, as my honey said, I was forced into a fast to save my life.

I encourage you to take the plunge before it's too late. Change your lifestyle and save your life. It is a matter of life or death.

Fasting

I would like to touch on a very powerful healing tool: fasting. I grew up in the evangelical church where fasting was a regular way of living. Every Wednesday my church held a fast for 24 hours. During that time, the adults fasted on water alone for

24 hours. Some did what's called a *dry fast* where they had nothing to drink nor eat.

I always felt that fasting was too hard and that I would never be able to do it. When I became ill in 2012, I was forced to fast. Like I mentioned before, Publix purified water is the only thing that did not make me deathly sick. It was after my divorce that I had started experimenting with fasting as I sought God's help. It was hard, but I stuck to a regular 24 hour fast every Tuesday. I found it easier to fast while at work because work took my mind off the hunger. Eventually, I didn't feel the need to continue, so I stopped. Years after, as I read, studied and researched, yearning to understand the formula for health and wellness, the formula to healing, I bumped into fasting as a way to health.

We all fast. Every night when we go to sleep, as we abstain from food and fluids, we fast. It is during this fasting that the cells, tissues, organs repair and heal themselves. When we eat and drink, our bodies are taking in nutrition. When we stop eating, when we fast, our bodies repair and heal themselves. Fasting leads to clear mindedness, reduced inflammation, weight loss, better control of blood glucose, increased energy, and better overall health. Fasting has been used for thousands of years to heal the body and strengthen the mind.

There are various types of fasts: *dry fast* means nothing by mouth. No foods, no liquids. *Intermittent fasting* is abstaining from foods for a specific length of time. An example of intermittent fasting is nothing to eat or drink for 12 hours per day. One can also fast on a specific diet for a specific time. I've done oatmeal and ripe banana fasts for 7 days and felt great as well as losing weight.

A very powerful detox fast that is not difficult at all is the *fruit fast.* Grapes, apples, lime, lemon, and grapefruit are wonderful for fruit fasts. This combination detoxes the body, and you won't feel like you're starving because the fruits makes you feel full and satisfied. You'll lose weight, and you'll be more clear-minded and energetic. I usually do this for at least 10 days to get the maximum effect. I recommend that you drink lots of water and herbal teas while fasting. Ginger and turmeric teas are great while fasting.

Why exercise?

Exercise and physical activity will lead to better health and is one of the tools to help to reduce the risk of developing diseases such as hypertension, heart disease, depression, sleep disorder, diabetes, cancer, obesity, and breathing problems like asthma. Obesity is a leading cause of death in the United States and the world at large. Walking is one of the best forms of exercise and is free. There is no need to pay money to join a gym. You only need to find a place where you can safely walk for at least 30 minutes per day for at least 4 days per week. If you can't do that, there are free exercise classes online that you can do in the comfort of your home. Hippocrates, who is called the father of western medicine, says walking is man's best medicine.

Walking

Walking helps to control and manage weight. Walking energizes and strengthens as it improves oxygenation to the organs, making us more clear-minded. Walking boosts the immune system. It reduces anxiety and stress, reduces blood pressure and blood sugar, and helps to stave off diseases and disorders. Oxygen supply to the organs is improved with walking and this will lead to healthier organs and a healthier overall body.

Walking healed my weak heart muscle, improving my ejection fraction from 35% to 65% in a very short few months. Walking is indeed a medicine without side effects.

Learn to be Still

Our state of mind contributes greatly to our overall health. I spend a lot of time in quietness and silence. Many call this meditation or prayer. Learn to be still. Be quiet. Take a walk by yourself. Sit outside by yourself. Be comfortable with your own company.

Once we learn to enjoy our own company, we will attain a sense of peace and tranquility. People who suffer from chronic states of anxiety, stress, worry, frustration, and fear tend to eat more unhealthy foods. They usually do not have a regular exercise schedule. Also, they do not sleep well as the busy mind keeps them awake at night or prevents them from falling asleep easily. All of this leads to the release of stress hormones, inflammation, and an overall unhealthy body, mind, and spirit.

Why sleep?

Many of us ignore the importance of sleep. I like to say that many people do not respect sleep. Not just any sleep but good quality and quantity sleep are vital to good health. It is while we sleep that our cells and tissues repair and heal themselves. As we get into a deep sleep, our blood pressure drops, heart rate drops, breathing slows and becomes regular and rhythmic. Adequate sleep helps to regulate our hormones, leading to better control of blood sugar. It also helps to boost our immunity. When properly rested, we tend to eat less food in general. We also tend to eat more nutritious foods when properly rested. Adequate sleep leads to clear-mindedness, and we are then able to think clearer and have a better memory. There has been much talk in recent years about the importance of sleep, adequate sleep. I feel fully rested when I get eight hours or more of sleep per night.

Insufficient quality and quantity of sleep affect every aspect of our lives. We become more forgetful and have what's called a foggy brain. We lack focus and are unable to concentrate. It can also cause us to have speech problems as we stutter and fumble with words. I've experienced these symptoms myself whenever I am sleep deprived.

Symptoms of Inadequate Sleep

- depression
- anxiety
- hopeless feelings
- feelings of doom
- fear
- nervousness
- shakiness
- headaches
- high blood pressure
- fast heart rate
- rapid breathing
- shortness of breath
- puffy eyes
- bags under the eyes
- dry, unhealthy looking skin
- constipation or diarrhea
- unsteady gait
- decreased immune system
- uncontrolled blood sugar

I do realize that some people can function quite well with less, however much research has been done in recent years where eight hours or more is recommended. Sleep affects the way we feel, our performance, and how we function in our daily activities. Undoubtedly, adequate sleep leads to an overall healthier state of health. My recommendation is to go to bed no later than eleven pm (preferably between 9pm and 10pm).

My personal experience has been that if I go to bed later than 11 pm and get the same 8 hours of sleep, I do not feel as well-rested as I would when I go to bed between 9 pm and 10 pm.

Why minimum stress level?

There has been so much talk about stress in recent years that I think that most people know by now how detrimental stress is to our overall health. Stress is unavoidable, that we know. The trick is to minimize the amount, minimize the level of stress.

I have heard it said that most heart attacks happen Monday mornings when folks are heading back to work after a short weekend off. That I do understand. I used to get anxious when returning to work after my days off until I realized the negative effects this was having on my mental, emotional, and physical health. This awareness helped me to learn to minimize the effects of stressors in my life.

Excessive stress can lead to

- low immunity
- anxiety
- depression
- suicidal thoughts
- fear
- irritability
- inability to sleep
- headaches
- trouble focusing and concentrating
- heart diseases like hypertension, palpitations, risk of a heart attack
- breathing problems
- hormonal imbalances
- constipation
- heartburn
- weight loss or weight gain
- irregular blood sugar
- overeating or under-eating

- eating unhealthy junk foods
- body pains
- tension
- fertility issues.

Excess stress also makes us look older and ages us. The list goes on.

We all get stressed out at times. That's to be expected. So much going on all the time. So many people clamoring for our attention. It's maddening. Stop! Take your time back. Say no! Learn to prioritize. Learn to relax and take time for yourself. Find a hobby, something you love and enjoy doing. Gardening, a sport, taking walks or going for a jog. Join the gym. Read, join a book club. Write a book, journal. Start a new business. Learn a new skill. Volunteer to help the needy, to read to kids, or at a nursing home to read to the elderly. Learn a musical instrument. Fishing is quite relaxing.

Spend time by yourself daily. Be still. You don't have to be busy all the time. Learn to chill. Have a routine. Go to bed at about the same time and wake up at about the same time. Have a winding-down time at night before going to sleep. This winding-down time should be quiet by yourself not in front of a television, Internet, phone, or any other device. Read something light and fun before going to sleep. Write 10 things for which you are grateful in your journal during this winding-down time.

It is very possible to live a low-stress life despite the constant hustle and bustle around us, but we must be intentional about it. Don't feel guilty about saying no and ignore those late phone calls from the drama friend or family member. It's your health, take charge of it.

THE HEALTHY PATH

Health is not only about food; health is more than just about what we eat. Health is about wholeness, which involves a healthy choice of foods, small portions of healthy foods, moderate exercise, walking at least 30 minutes at least four days per week, minimum stress and at least eight hours of good restful sleep per night.

When these are done regularly, you will begin to feel alive, strong, energetic, and happy. Hippocrates, who is called the father of western medicine stated, "Your food is your medicine and your medicine is your food." He also stated, "If you are not your doctor, you are a fool." He also advises that "walking is man's best medicine."

We are in the middle of a coronavirus/ Covid19 pandemic where over 135,000 persons have died with over 30,000 in New York City alone in less than four months. The data to date indicates that the ones with the highest mortality are those with preexisting conditions of hypertension, diabetes, obesity, coronary heart disease, kidney disease, hypercholesterolemia, asthma, and dementia, or preexisting conditions that were not officially diagnosed by a physician. 55% of those who died had hypertension. 37% had diabetes. This statistic makes me very angry as I know that, for the most part, these disease conditions are very preventable.

The United States has some of the most obese and overweight people in the world. With this obesity comes a myriad of health problems. The solution it seems, to all our ills, are pills and injections. There is a pill for everything, it seems. As the media begins to show pictures of the younger deceased, I notice that there is a trend. They're obese. Young in age but old in health.

With obesity comes hypertension, diabetes, asthma, kidney disease, heart diseases and high cholesterol, and for the most parts, these are the underlying conditions that have led to the very poor outcomes of those that have succumbed to this deadly virus.

Although Covid19 is a very deadly infection, we must remember that many thousands of people die each year from the flu. The most vulnerable are always those with compromised immunity, and these are usually in the groups mentioned above. There needs to be a wholistic approach to health and wellness. I believe that the Department of Health needs to be responsible for providing adequate preventative healthcare and educating the public at large about proper nutrition and exercise. Junk food is often cheaper than healthier foods, so folks tend to choose junk rather than healthy foods. The Health Department needs to ensure that fruits, vegetables, nuts, seeds, and grains are affordable for all.

One of the first things we were taught in nursing school was handwashing. We learned that handwashing is the single most effective way to prevent the spread of infections. Isn't this something that the Department of Health ought to be teaching children and adults alike? Why did they have to wait till Covid19?

We as individuals and family units need to also take responsibility for our health by making healthy dietary choices, eating less and incorporating moderate exercises for the entire family as part of our daily regimen. Families and friends can incorporate fun activities to do together. Parents and other responsible adults can teach the younger ones by example to make rest, relaxation and sleep a priority. It's a matter of life or death. I do believe that if we were healthier, yes, Covid19 might still infect us; however, our bodies would be strong and resilient enough to fight and overcome it. Only the strongest survive is a popular saying and it is true.

Now, I also hear many talks of the FDA expeditiously approving an antiviral drug to treat the sickest Covid19 patients. Pharmaceutical companies are working night and day in their pursuit to be the one to make the long talked about Covid19 vaccine. Why am I not surprised by this? This too is about cashing in, about the almighty dollar, as they say.

Like I said, everything that ails us has a drug to treat without much thought into the many potentially deadly side effects. Did I mention that tens of thousands of people die every year from drug adverse reactions? Perhaps more than the coronavirus. Healthcare is big business here in the United States and many other countries. The healthcare industry does not want us to be healthy. How could they make the multi-million dollars if we are healthy?

The cycle is to keep us busy, so we have no time to exercise, no time to cook healthy meals, no time to sleep, no time to rest, no time for fun. We grab junk and fast food as we dash to and from work. There are fast food joints everywhere, and they're constantly advertising to tempt us. Fried, super-sized, sweet junk. Salty junk. That's what we eat for breakfast, lunch and dinner plus in between. We're getting fatter and fatter by the day and no one has the guts to tell us as we eat ourselves to death. Children, teenagers, young adults, middle-aged and older adults are so overweight and sick. Why? Because of our diet, lack of exercise, insufficient sleep and excess stress.

Let's take back what rightfully belongs to us, our health. Our physical, emotional, and spiritual health!

Sample of my daily Healthy Path

- Wake up at 6:30 am.
- Do a few stretches while in bed.
- Pray: "Thank you God for a new day. Thank you for life, health and strength, peace of mind, joy, happiness

and contentment. It is a new day, and I'm so grateful to be alive. Amen." This is my daily mantra and prayer every day.

- Drink eight ounces of warm water with a slice of lemon. This helps to keep my bowel regular. Sometimes I add a dropper -full of cayenne tincture which helps to energize and jump start my day.

- A cup of coffee or herbal tea while I relax under my favorite tree watching the birds. This is a form of meditation.

- Walk for 2 to 3 miles at a brisk, steady pace. The pace should be so that one can hold a conversation without getting out of breath. I will sometimes do a slow jog for a bit. While exercising, I sip on 16 ounces of water. Our bodies are made up of more than 60% water, so it is very important to drink enough water so that we do not get dehydrated. I believe that our bodies need at least 6 to 8 eight-ounce glasses of water per day to stay hydrated and healthy. That is 48 to 64 ounces of water per day.

- After exercising, I boil a 4-ounce cup of old-fashioned oatmeal with 1 tablespoon of a mix of flax seeds, chia seeds, and hemp seeds. Quick oatmeal is not the best and can cause constipation, so I stay away from quick oatmeal. Add fruits to this, usually one ripe banana or half an apple, a handful of berries or a slice of pineapple. Sometimes one tablespoon of raisins, a pinch of cinnamon and nutmeg and one teaspoon of moringa powder. I have tried skipping breakfast but found that it made me very lightheaded and also caused me to overeat at dinner if I didn't have a healthy breakfast. This is what I eat for breakfast every day. The fruit varies.

- I never eat lunch. Dinner time is between 3 pm and 4 pm. Here is a typical dinner meal for us: during the warmer months we eat salad every day. This usually includes celery, parsley, broccoli, cucumber, tomatoes, raw onion, raw garlic, avocado and wild plants in our yard. Salad dressing is a little olive oil with apple cider vinegar. Sautéed beans or peas. I cook my peas and beans from scratch. Usually, cooking at least one pound and stick it in the refrigerator sautéing as needed. Starch is usually sweet potatoes, wild rice, quinoa, and squashes. Between breakfast and dinner, I will eat fruits or just drink water.

- Later if I feel a little hungry, I usually have a cup of herbal teas and a fruit. Throughout the day sipping on room temperature water. It is not good to drink cold water as it shocks our organs. While growing up, I always saw the older folks drinking warm or room temperature water. The United States is one of the few countries where people have so much ice-cold water. While vacationing in Italy, my friend requested ice for her mineral water. The waiter looked at her as if to say "That's weird. The water is already cold." As a rule of thumb, if you're urinating often, and the urine is nice and clear or a pale yellow, it's usually a pretty good indication that you're drinking enough water. If you're experiencing thirst, you are already dehydrated; drink up!

- After cleaning up my kitchen, I relax with a book, hang out with my family, do some writing, or something that I like to do. Take a stroll in my garden, walk my dog. It's very important to do some things that you like. This will make you happy and content. Find a hobby, something that makes you feel good. Do something to help others. This will take the focus off just yourself and make you feel fulfilled and purposeful, leading to joy, contentment, and peace of mind.

- Bedtime is between 9 pm and 10 pm every night. It's very healthy to have a bedtime routine. If you do, your body will automatically tell you when it's time to go to bed without having to set a timer or to even look at a clock. When you sleep better and get good quality sleep (about 8 hours), this will lead to a healthier you. You will wake up feeling rested and ready for the day's challenge. Another thing is to refrain from checking your emails close to bedtime and dim the lights in your house.

Herbal (Bush)Teas

As a child growing up in Jamaica West Indies, the herbs (aka bush) were widely used to heal and cure all kinds of illnesses. Headaches, menstrual cramps, infertility, toothaches, joint pains, inflammation, and high blood pressure are just a few of the conditions that the "bush doctor" would treat. These worked, and folks knew which bush to take for their specific condition. The bush doctor was well respected, and very few went to a conventional doctor when they were sick. It was common to see people live to be well into their 80s and 90s and even 100s, strong and independent.

As people all over the world turn to drugs to treat their ailments, they might live long, but they are weak with one foot in the grave and one out. Prescription and over the counter drugs come with so many bad side effects. They are supposed to help us with one thing, but they eventually cause so many other ailments; we wonder why we ever took them in the first place. Have you read the side effects of these so-called medications recently?

Herbal teas are chock full of nutrients and wonderful antioxidants. They are relaxing and healing. My dad is 88 years old, and he swears that bush teas (aka herbal teas) have kept him healthy for this long. Part of his nightly regimen is to have a mug of bush tea. His favorite combination consists of cerrassee, mint and guinea hen weed boiled for 20 minutes, and he always makes enough to last a few days. He adds some cinnamon powder and sweetens the tea with a bit of honey.

My dad is very healthy and independent. He washes his clothes by hand and hangs them on a clothesline in the sun. He irons them himself. He cleans and cooks for himself every day. Conducts his own business. He has had enlarged prostate for over 50 years and believes that guinea hen weed teas have prevented his prostates from becoming cancerous. There has been research done and many testimonials about the anticancer properties of guinea hen weed.

My mom is 84 years old, and the only health issue she has is, as she calls it, "a touch of high blood pressure." Mom is very strong, healthy and clear minded. She eats mainly plant-based foods and very little meat as she cannot afford to buy much meat. She has always been a walker and goes to bed by 9 pm every night. Mom loves to laugh and is surrounded by her grandchildren who bring joy to her living.

I too have incorporated a hot cup of herbal/ bush teas to my daily regimen. I like to experiment with different bushes and herbs: fennel seeds, caraway seeds, ginger roots, turmeric root, moringa leaves, soursop leaves, cerasee leaves, mints, dandelion flowers, roots, and leaves, and pomegranate leaves are just a few to choose from.

I usually boil at least 4 of the above together in a large pot for 20 minutes. Leave overnight. Reheat an 8 oz mug of it each evening and sip on it as I relax at the end of the day.

Bush Tea Recipes

This tea is excellent for sleep and relaxation

- 2 dried or green soursop leaves
- 1 handful of dried moringa leaves
- Mint of choice
- Mashed or grated ginger root
- 4 cups water

Makes 4 cups of tea.

Bring water to boil. Add all the ingredients. Lower heat to low. Boil for 20 minutes.

Sweeten with a little organic raw honey (optional). When the liquid is cool, stick the pot with the ingredients in the water into the refrigerator. Strain and reheat just the amount you plan to drink each time. Enjoy!

This tea is great for inflammation.

It has helped my body to rid itself of arthritis, joint and muscle pain and soreness.

- Turmeric root (mashed or grated)
- Dandelion root

Boil together for 20 minutes. Turn off heat and let sit in water until cool. Place the pot in the refrigerator. When ready to drink, just reheat the amount you need.

Add a bit of raw organic honey to taste. Honey is a natural anti-inflammatory food.

RECIPES

One of the delights of cooking is learning to cook simply. By doing so one can enjoy the taste of the individual food and its spices. Here's an example:

Sautéed lentils

Delicious, easy, and healthy. Any bean can be cooked and sautéed with any spice we desire. I often use chickpeas, black beans, red beans, and lentils.

Wash lentils. Remove any rocks or debris. Cook until tender, not mushy. Strain and discard water.

- 1 medium onion, chopped
- 1 medium tomato, chopped
- 4 cloves fresh garlic, minced
- Fresh or dried rosemary, thyme or mint to taste
- Fennel seeds 1/2 tsp

In a saucepan add oil of your choice. I like to cook with coconut or olive oils. Bring to heat. Add the onion, garlic, tomato, and rosemary/thyme/mint. Stir.

Add ground red pepper, fennel seeds & seasoning salt/sea salt. Stir. Sauté on low heat for about 5 minutes. Stir in the lentils. Cover and simmer for another 5 minutes. Serve with a salad, steamed vegetables or rice.

Fresh raw vegetable salad

- Fresh parsley washed
- Broccoli florets
- 1 ripe tomato

- 1 slice onion finely minced
- 1 clove fresh garlic finely minced
- 1 ripe hass avocado
- 1 stalk celery
- 1/2 cucumber

Cut all the vegetables into small pieces. place in a bowl. Drizzle with raw organic apple cider vinegar.

Optional:

- add cooked quinoa, wild rice, brown rice.
- add fruits like chopped apples, pineapple.
- add nuts, beans, peas.

These will add flavor to your salad and make it more filling.

Digestive herbal teas

This tea is excellent for flatus/excess gas, heartburn, bloating. The ingredients have anti-inflammatory properties and antioxidants that may help to treat or prevent cancer and heart disease. This tea is a pain reliever and also helps with sleep.

- Fresh organic ginger root mashed or grated
- Fresh organic turmeric root mashed or grated
- Fennel seeds and or caraway seeds
- Mint of choice

Bring water to boil in a pot and add the above ingredients, Turn heat down to low. Boil on low for 20 minutes. Turn off heat and let it brew for 2 hours. Sweeten with raw organic honey to taste [optional].

This makes enough to last for about 3 days, reheat just the needed amount each time. Stick the pot with the leftover tea into the fridge and reheat the portion you intend to drink as needed.

I drink this tea frequently as beans and peas are part of my daily diet. Like most people, I have difficulty digesting legumes. This tea helps a lot. I also cook with these ingredients. This tea was a lifesaver for me during the years of early menopause when I suffered from severe gastric issues like bloating, excess gas, constipation, trapped abdominal gas, heartburn, and acid reflux.

Quinoa and rice

- 1 cup multicolored quinoa
- 1 cup wild rice
- salt to taste
- 1 slice onion minced
- 1 clove fresh garlic minced
- 1/4 teaspoon fresh or dried rosemary leaves
- 1 whole red hot pepper (do not cut)
- 1 teaspoon coconut oil
- 3 whole cloves
- 3 whole pimento
- 4 cups water

Wash rice and quinoa. Drain off water. Bring water to boil and add all the ingredients except the whole pepper. Stir. Bring to boil on medium heat. Stir in whole pepper. Turn down heat to low. Cover and let cook. Turn heat to simmer when most of the water is absorbed. Let simmer till cooked.

Wild rice takes longer to cook than cheap rice; however, wild rice is the best rice to eat and is well worth spending a little more to buy if you're serious about healthy eating. Wild rice is rich in many nutrients such as potassium, carbohydrate, dietary fiber, protein calcium, iron, and magnesium.

Curried Chickpeas

This is the less healthy version that I would do if I were cooking for a party of meat lovers.

It is best to cook your beans and peas from scratch to avoid the extra salt and additives which are bad for us.

Soak peas or beans overnight in the refrigerator. Pour off the water the next morning and cook with fresh water. I have a pressure cooker which will cook most dried beans in 30 minutes.

- 1 pound cooked chickpeas (save 1/4 cup of the juice)
- 1/2 green, yellow and red sweet peppers cut into small pieces
- 1 scotch bonnet or spicy red pepper cut finely
- 1 green scotch bonnet pepper whole
- 1 tablespoon dried or green thyme leaves
- 1 large ripe tomato cut small
- 1 medium onion cut small
- 3 large cloves fresh garlic minced finely
- 1 large carrot cut thin lengthwise
- 1 medium sweet potato washed and cut into small cubes
- 2 slices pumpkin chopped into small pieces
- 1 stick butter
- seasoning salt to taste
- black pepper to taste
- 1/2 tsp cumin powder
- 2 slices fresh ginger root cut into tiny pieces
- 1/2 tsp powdered allspice
- 1/4 tsp fennel seed
- 1/4 tsp caraway seeds
- 1/4 cup coconut milk
- 1/4 cup cooking oil of choice
- 6 tablespoon spicy curry powder

Place pot on stove over medium heat. Add oil and butter. When butter is melted and oil is hot, add curry and stir for 2 minutes. Stir in all vegetables and spices except whole pepper. Add coconut milk and stir well. Add cooked chickpeas and the 1/4 cup of chickpeas juice. Stir well. Throw in whole green scotch bonnet pepper. Cover and simmer till carrots and pumpkin are tender.

Serve with rice, quinoa, salad or your favorite dish.

YOUR NEXT STEPS

Helping Yourself

Here is a summary of how you can get on and stay on a healthy path to attain and maintain an overall healthy lifestyle:

- Adopt a primarily plant-based diet. Fruits, vegetables, nuts, seeds, grains.
- Flesh or meat should be rare.
- Never eat processed meat like salami, ham, sausages etc.
- Gradually switch to plant-based foods by eliminating meats and flesh one day per week for one month. For example, meatless Fridays. Then increase to two days for one month and so on until you've cut out animal products completely from your diet.
- Eat beans/peas every day. They are cheap, easy and loaded with nutrients including protein, calcium, iron. Cook your beans and peas with ginger root and fennel seeds for easier digestion.
- Be creative with your cooking to make your plant-based foods enjoyable and delicious as you would with meats and flesh.
- Drink 6 to 8 glasses of water each day.
- Exercise at least 4 days per week for at least 30 minutes each day. Walking is the best exercise and it is free.

- Try to get 7 to 8 hours of sleep every night. Go to bed at the same time every night. Our bodies heal and repair itself during sleep. A good night's sleep helps us to wake up in a good mood, feeling refreshed and ready to face the day's challenges.

- Prayer and meditation are a must. Spend at least 15 minutes in quiet time by yourself. Journal, expressing gratitude for the things that are going well for you. Prayer, meditation, quiet time heals the soul and leads to contentment, joy, happiness, peace of mind and a settled spirit.

- Find a hobby or something you love and do it. This will give you purpose and a sense of accomplishment. Help others that are less fortunate than yourself.

- Maintain a positive mindset. Use the 'I am' mantra (positive affirmations). E.g. *I am strong. I am beautiful. I am able.*

- Ask a friend or family member to hold you accountable for the choices you make.

- Have a health buddy. Iron sharpens iron. We help each other.

- Adopt a pet if you're lonely.

What if you are doing the best you can to take great care of your overall health. What if your loved ones struggle or have many difficulties following the above guidelines I've outlined in this book.

How, you might ask, can I help my best friend, my sister, my brother, my spouse, my children?

How might I help them if they're stubborn and won't listen or if they just don't know how to go about it.

Many people have no clue how to start a healthy protocol. It's not about being academically educated. Many have degrees but are clueless about healthy living, it's not taught in schools and healthcare. It's nothing to be ashamed of.

My question to you is - what if you knew that these folks that you love so much have cancer, and you knew for sure that there was a cure, would you tell them about that cure and just leave them alone? Or would you tell them and keep telling and encouraging them to give that cure a try?

I recall when a famous lady died from supposedly drug problems. I heard many people say that if she were their loved ones they would have broken down her gated community wall, kicked her door in, and dragged her to a drug rehabilitation center.

Woulda coulda shoulda! Everybody likes to say, " I wish I had..."

I know that my loved ones may often get tired of me as I push, encourage, educate, and remind them constantly to take the best care of themselves. To quit smoking. To drink a minimum of 6 glasses of water daily, shoot for 8 glasses. To walk, to turn off the television, to get some zzz's!

Helping Others

I feel it's my responsibility to push, encourage, and remind them that their health is their wealth. This is what the Bible means by being our brother's keeper. Nagging doesn't help. A gentle push does, a reminder that I love them and want them around healthy and strong for a long time usually works.

- You can hand that child or your partner a bottle of water even if they haven't asked you to.
- You can pick up that friend or family member and take them to the park to walk with you.

- You can express lovingly your concern about them smoking, eating unhealthy food, not exercising enough.

- You can decide not to call them late at night as you set the example of going to bed early and getting adequate sleep which contributes to health and wellness.

- You can share healthy recipes with them.

- You can help the children and your partner; you can take walks as a family.

- You can get involved in a sport as a family.

- You can buy healthy and cook healthy foods for the family.

- You can offer the children fruits and vegetables for snacks instead of cookies.

- You can choose to have no soda and no so-called juice in your household.

- You can make your fruit juice from scratch and teach the children to do so also. So-called juice should never be offered to children unless you make it from scratch yourself. Store-bought so-called juices have sugar and other preservatives that are bad for human consumption and addictive.

- You can introduce vegetables and fruits to the children and grandchildren as soon as they start solids. They'll acquire the taste for them.

- You can offer infants water as soon as the pediatrician gives the okay, so that they grow up to love water, the tasteless colorless drink that is more than 60% of our body, that is vital for living.

- You can choose to remove junk food from your home. I was not a nurse when my children were born, but I knew enough to decide that I did not want any, or at least much, junk food in my home. I did the best I knew then to prepare healthy meals for my family. I did not offer my children cookies except on rare occasions like birthday parties. No sodas could be found in my refrigerator. I wish I knew then what I know now, my choices would have been much better.

TALK, TALK, TALK to your loved ones. Taking their hands and gently leading is one way. One day they'll thank you. Not everyone changes quickly or overnight. Keep the conversation going and keep encouraging. The Christian Bible states that we are our brother's keeper. We are all brothers and sisters. Let's not give up on anyone if they're not changing the habits when we want them to.

People change every day. My part, your part is to support, remind, and keep encouraging them to change to a healthier lifestyle. If you find yourself getting too pushy about the matter, back off and change strategies. I find that people do remember when we teach them what to do to attain and maintain great health, but they might not be quite ready yet.

Another strategy is to modify our expectations of lifestyle changes. Instead of asking them to exercise every day for 45 minutes, we can suggest 4 days per week for 30 minutes or even break up the 30 minutes into 3 ten minutes intervals. Be creative in your approach.

Help by being the example. It is said that children learn by example, so do adults. When you go out to lunch, breakfast, dinner with friends or family, make a healthier choice. They'll take note even if nothing is said.

When I go to the grocery store there is always someone who asks or comments on the fact that I have only vegetables, fruits, nuts, grains, and no animal products in my shopping cart. It is always a perfect opportunity for me to start a conversation about plant-based eating, how sick I was a few years ago, and how lifestyle changes led to my current healthy state. I also quickly mention how easy it is to transition to plant-based eating and I can't help but boast a tiny bit about how disease free I am at 58 years of age and on no drugs. They are always surprised.

I find that many think that plant-based eating means eating boring salads for breakfast, lunch, and dinner. I'm often asked how I prepare beans, for example. This is another opportunity to educate.

Well, if our loved ones are sick due to poor lifestyle choices, let's do what we need to do over and over and over again. Perhaps they will eventually listen, and you'll save them.

On a last note, if you're feeling low on energy, if you're just dragging yourself around, having to push yourself to get through the day, if your brain is foggy and you're often forgetful, go down the list and check off each category that I've named:

1. How is your nutrition?

2. How is your exercise & activity?

3. How is your sleep?

4. How is your stress level?

I guarantee that it is most likely one of these that is off. That needs to be addressed and adjusted. Sometimes it's as simple as **drinking more water**.

Our health is our responsibility.

Take the best care of it!

Eat, Sleep, Mediate!

ABOUT THE AUTHOR

Marva Riley has been a registered nurse for over twenty years. She is also the recipient of The Daisy Award for Extraordinary Nurses, honoring nurses internationally. Most of her experience has been in critical care. She is an educator and believes that we are all educators in our own rights, that it is everyone's responsibility to teach others what we know to be true.

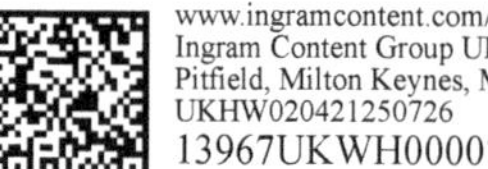
www.ingramcontent.com/pod-product-compliance
Ingram Content Group UK Ltd.
Pitfield, Milton Keynes, MK11 3LW, UK
UKHW020421250726
13967UKWH00007B/2761

9 780578 728070